How to Walk Correctly

Empowering
yourself to solve

Low Back Pain
Shin Splints
Sciatica
Plantar Fasciitis
Falling Arches
Knee Pain
Scoliosis
and any other leg issues

Written and Illustrated by
Jacob Caldwell, LMP

How to Walk Correctly

Empowering yourself to Solve

Low Back Pain
Shin Splints
Sciatica
Plantar Fasciitis
Falling Arches
Knee Pain
Scoliosis
and any other leg issues

Written & Illustrated

By

Jacob Caldwell, LMP

Copyright 2011-2018

Introduction

Empower your health with knowledge and solve your own ailments.

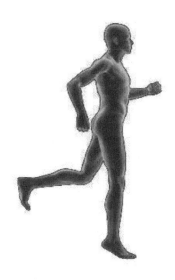

WARNING: The Walking Series is for people who want to empower their own self-healing and take control of their life. Do not read any further if you have a closed mind and are looking for excuses as to why you are not getting better. Without an open mind, upcoming text may be very disturbing and frightening to you. If one reads and carries out these techniques you may become healthier, happier, and not have any more excuses to use. The Walking Series is for Perseverant and Personally Responsible People only. You have been Warned! Good Luck!

"How to Walk Correctly", is so simple of a statement it doesn't make sense. "Of course, I know how to walk; I've been doing it since I was born." Yes, you have been. What we have also could have been doing is creating chronic inflammatory ailments at the same time by not walking correctly. In sports, technique will win out over strength most of the time.

As a Massage Therapist, my focus and passion has always been to empower people to heal themselves. Healer means

"To Inspire", Doctor means "To Teach", and in my book if you are not being taught or inspired by your practitioner on how to resolve your issue, then this is called Failure. Failure in medicine and therapy is when you repeat the same practice and achieve very little progress with the same level of pain for the client. The same definition applies to "Insanity" – doing the same thing over and over again and expecting a different result.

I have always been curious on how an injury occurs. It always seems like a game to me in finding the mystery to how the pain got there. Often many people do not know what the source of their pain is and usually practitioners don't bother to find out. It is imperative to find out how that hip pain got there. Was it from a fall 10 years ago or is it from walking your dog every day? If we can prevent an incorrect activity that is causing us pain, then we can administer the correct healing procedure. However, we need the person to stop hurting themselves so that they can progressively heal. If the person is currently hurting themselves on a daily basis it is quite difficult to have an effective treatment plan.

The most profound and preventable injury that I see is that people do not walk correctly. As a society, we don't really walk anymore. We walk to the bathroom, to the car, down the hall, but now we rarely walk a mile or 2 to work or to the store. Sometimes I will hear, "I had to park 3 blocks away to get here!" If you have trouble walking 3 blocks, you need to walk those 3 blocks. We are such a technological society that we have stomped on Nature for egotistical technology. We think a MRI and surgery is going to help us with our knee issue when really it comes to flexing a muscle correctly. We think technology is going to save us from everything, but if we can listen to Nature it has all the solutions already. The problem is we must listen to Nature and accept things are easy, which is the hard part.

I have seen many different pain issues such as Arthritis, Scoliosis, Plantar Fasciitis, Bursitis, inflamed joints, ACL/MCL tears, shin splints, falling arches, tight IT Bands, bunions, low back pain, chronic neck pain, and one leg shorter than the other. As far as I am concerned these issues all must do with one thing: HOW YOUR FOOT CONTACTS THE GROUND. If you have ever constructed a house you would know that the leveling of the foundation is an important part of the building process, otherwise you will have crooked windows, walls, and roofs. So, goes the same with the body.

The full range of motion of the leg and foot must be exercised; otherwise, if one continually skips parts of the steps it will be like a house on a slowly sinking foundation. Soon you will have chronic issues above the waist and no matter what kind of therapy you do, the issue never resolves and continually reappears. Usually where the pain is, is not the problem, but the symptom. If the window is crooked it has nothing to do with the window itself; it is the crooked foundation and the same thing happens with the body. Often crooked hips and low back pain must do with the simple technique of not flexing your big toe. You can rub that back all you want but if you do not flex that toe, your back is going to keep hurting for a long time.

There have been many devices like orthotics, ointments, and surgeries but all of these are temporary solutions. If you do not flex that foot correctly nothing will change. I have had people lay on my massage bed and they think all they need is for me to rub that spot and it will be gone. And then I have to apologize and say, "This session is only effective for inspiring you on how to heal" and "you sir/ma'am need to flex your foot properly."

Unfortunately, walking correctly is not an easy thing to master at first and takes a lot of discipline. Breaking habits is very difficult but the rewards to being able to heal yourself and prevent further injury are quite empowering. I like to think, if I was thrown out into the forest, would I have to need anything? I don't want to have to depend on needing something like pharmaceuticals, orthotics, or syringes. I want to be truly health empowered with self-knowledge. After learning the "Walking Correct Technique" you are going to have to ask yourself, "If I can heal this what else can I do?" Answer: Everything!

At first, learning how to walk again requires a lot of thinking about your feet and can seem overwhelming and that is why I have broken the steps up so that you can focus on one thing at a time. It is tough to do them all at once but if you can do one, you can do the next.

Chapter 1:

ROM of the Ankles is equal to ROM of the HIP

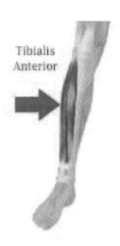

Tibialis
Anterior

Flexibility and excising the full ROM ("range of motion") of any appendage should be a major goal to focus on. This is what I like about yoga; it puts you in positions you would not ordinarily get into yourself. While yoga helps to tone and strengthen joints while utilizing full range of motion; the key to mastering the full 10-part Walking Series is to practice body awareness and foot presence.

I have observed that most people's ankles are stiff and are stuck at the 90-degree ankle. When the leg takes a step forward, the front of the foot should be lifted upwards as well, while making sure to hit the heel on the ground first and not be flat-footed. You should feel your Tibialis Anterior working very hard and if it hurts you are doing it right.

When you lift the foot an inch more upwards, this will allow your leg to move farther forward in its stride. People with hip issues and tight IT Bands often fall into this category. (IT Band is located on the outside of the leg between the knee and hip.) If one is NOT lifting their foot and allowing their leg to move forward you will be causing the front of your hip to become atrophied and stale. Staleness in a joint will become hard because blood circulation cannot move

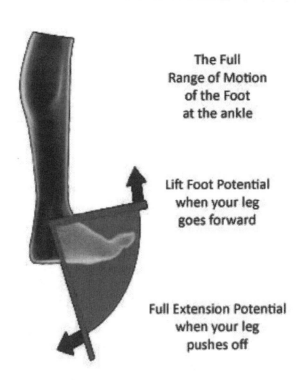

The Full
Range of Motion
of the Foot
at the ankle

Lift Foot Potential
when your leg
goes forward

Full Extension Potential
when your leg
pushes off

through the muscle. This will make your joint less maneuverable and may make it susceptible to being injured later. Tight muscles are like glass and if jarred suddenly they shatter. Having your muscles and joints lucid and flexible with a full range of motion will help keep them more tolerable to outer circumstances.

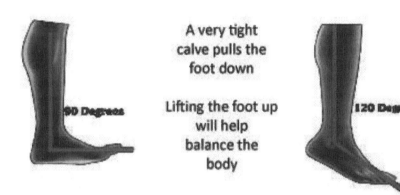

A very tight calve pulls the foot down

Lifting the foot up will help balance the body

It is good to massage your Tibialis Anterior to help loosen up the ankle. Hold the muscle and flex your foot up and down. Flex into the muscle while pressing into it. Continue to press into it while stretching it downwards. This is a bit of the StretchFlex Technique™, to be learned at the end of this book.

Chapter 2:

Toes Forward

In a full-length leg stride, it is imperative to have your toes pointed forward the whole time! It is easy to think you are doing this when your leg is in front of you. But what people miss is the technique when your leg is behind you. When your leg is behind you it is easy to turn your foot outwards. In my office I estimate about 80% of people will point their toes outwards and the other 20% will point their toes inwards.

Walking with your toes pointed inwards may lead to pains on the inside of the legs or front of the hips.

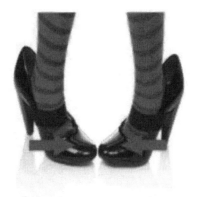
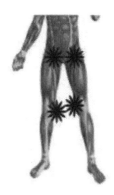

If you walk with your toes pointed outward you will be using more of the outside leg muscles. Like in Part 1, it is key to achieve full range of motion in all joints. If you are only using one side of your leg, this is where shin splints, hip issues and low back pain will develop later. People who have their toes pointed inwards will have plantar fasciitis, toe arthritis, and tight front hips.

Your hip muscles are in charge of changing direction when you are walking. Deep Tissue Massage and stretching these areas will help with improving toe direction. Sitting on a Yoga ball while flexing into the ball will help break up tight hip muscles.

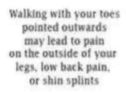

Walking with your toes pointed outwards may lead to pain on the outside of your legs, low back pain, or shin splints

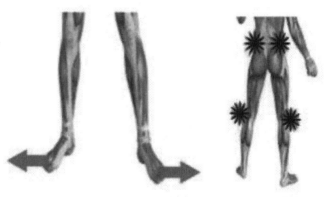

Start practicing walking with your toes pointed forward, to help you get ready for Part 3.

Take note to follow Walking Correctly Chapter 9 which will go in to detail on how your Mental Pattern creates which way your toes point.

Chapter 3:

The 4 Step Points

Now we get a little more detailed and break up the foot into 4 specific contact points.

Step Point 1: Heal

Step Point 2: Outside Ball of Foot

Step Point 3: Inside Ball of Foot

Step Point 4: Big Toe

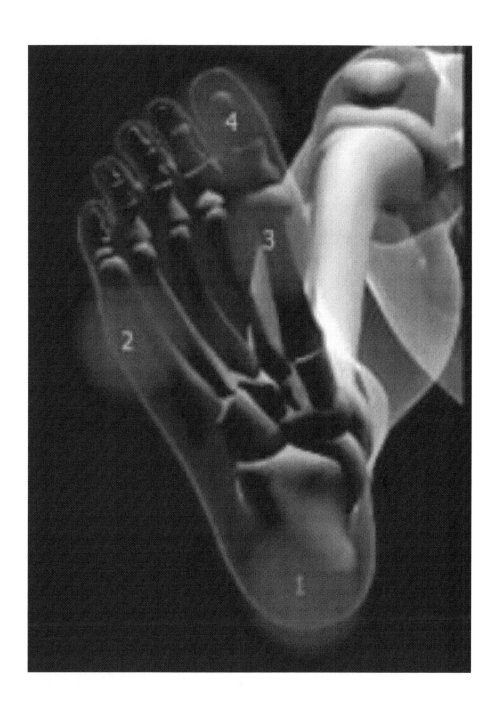

It is important to hit each point individually. Often outward pointed toe walkers will combine Step Points 3 and 4 together. This will lead to very tight outside IT Bands, shin splints, and low back pain. Inward pointed toe walkers will skip Step Point 1, which will lead to tight front hips.

It is important to hit Step Point 1 and 2 when your leg is in front of you. Step Point 3 and 4 occur when your leg is behind you.

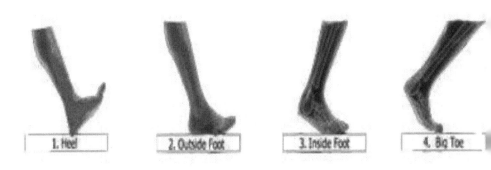

1. Heel   2. Outside Foot   3. Inside Foot   4. Big Toe

Also, take notice of the muscles in your legs while you're walking. When your leg is in front of you, you will use the outside leg muscles. When your leg is behind you, you are going to use your inside leg muscles.

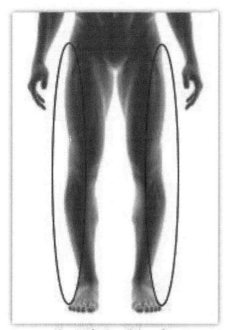

| Outside Leg Muscles | Inside Leg Muscles |

While you are walking, your feet should behave like a wave fluctuating from outside to inside, while rocking back and forth. However, to the observer, it will look like nothing is going on.

Tip: Use some deep tissue massage therapy on the inside arch of your foot.

Chapter 4:

Grip the Ground – No more Falling Arches

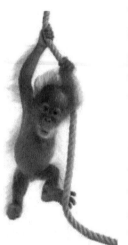

To keep the integrity of your arch, it is a requirement that you have good dexterity in your feet. Gripping the ground and resisting the pull of gravity is important.

In Part 3, between Step Point 2 & 3 is when you flex your outside foot to the inside foot. At this point is where you want to grip and squeeze the ground and feel yourself holding your body up. Falling arches are due to flaccid and sloppy foot technique which allows your feet to flop around. Strong feet will have strong arches. Plantar Fasciitis and Falling Arches can be prevented here. When practiced properly, this gripping and flexing technique can prevent extreme debilitating pain from occurring. With a little foot flexing, many of your foot pain issues will go away.

Tip: The StretchFlex™ Technique for your Arch - step on a tennis ball and massage the ball along your arch while flexing and stretching your foot. Suggested time on this exercise is just 2-5 minutes a day. After 1-2 weeks, the pain may be drastically reduced or gone.

Chapter 5:

Finesse – Relax, Spread, Flex, and Stretch

Now that you have worked on improving your range of motion and getting some flexibility in your feet, now it is easier to work on some more intricate helpful techniques.

Our muscles and joints work best when we can flex and stretch them to their full capacity. This is also very important with the feet. As a society we bind our feet in shoes that are either too tight or have too thick of a sole. Walking correctly really requires being able to feel the ground and squeeze the Earth below us. Our hands and feet have the same muscles; we should be just as strong in our feet as our hands.

It is important to master the beginning 1-4 Parts before being successful at this section.

1. When your leg is swinging forward, relax your foot and hit Step Point 1. Feel your foot spread out and open as wide as possible.

2. When you move toward Step Point 2 and 3 begin to flex your foot and really grip the ground.

3. When moving through Step Point 3 and 4 your foot will begin stretching to its full range of motion outward.

4. Follow through – Like in every sport, follow through is important. When your foot has left the ground keep pointing the toe inward and pointed and feel the full-length stride.

This part is important to feel the full range of your foot fully relaxed and fully flexed in every stride that you take.

Note: Most Yoga Instructors talk about "old age starts in the toes". When atrophy starts in your toes, the rigidness slowly goes up your body and your joints become like concrete. Each joint becomes less and less flexible.

Tip: Also getting a massage 1-2 times a month is best to counteract a full 40 hours a week sitting at your desk.

Chapter 6:

Walking Improves Health

The Path of the Spleen Meridian through the Arch of the Foot (pic. from AcuGraph).

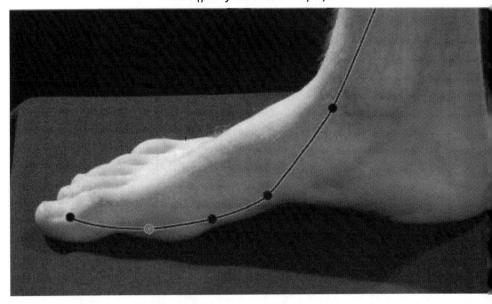

Immune System – Protects the Body

In Acupuncture, the meridian points in the fingers and toes are toning the corresponding organs. In the feet, the Meridians are the Spleen, Liver, Stomach, Gall Bladder, Bladder, and the Kidneys. These organs help with overall strength and the immune system. Each of the toning points of organs encircles all areas of the foot, so it is important to tone the muscles of the foot evenly. If a part of the foot is often skipped by lack of circulation and stimulation, that organ will have low energy or restricted flow making the organ "tired" or "sluggish".

So, walking correctly and excising the whole foot will increase overall energy and a stronger immune system.

Lymphatic System – Cleans the Body

In the circulation system, the heart is the muscle that moves the blood throughout the body. In the lymphatic system there is no singular system that moves the water throughout your body. The lymph's are in your arm pits, breasts, between the legs, and calves. When the surrounding muscles are flexed, this pumps water throughout the body. Walking is one of the best ways to circulate water throughout the body. Where there is circulation, there is healing and strength.

Tip: Massage is also a recommended way to support the lymphatic system. Squeezing muscles helps pump water through tight muscles.

Chapter 7:

Walking Incorrectly Affects Posture

One leg is shorter or longer than the other

Often when one leg is shorter than the other it is because that person leans on the shorter leg more than the other. They do this because in the past they have sprained or broken something on the opposite leg, and they will walk on the healthy leg to relieve pressure on the injured leg. After the injury heals, if they do not equally walk on both legs, they will continually lean on the "healthy leg".

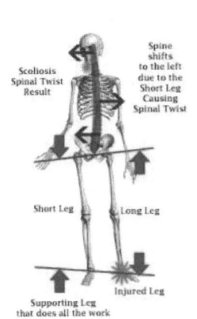

Spine shifts to the left due to the Short Leg Causing Spinal Twist

Scoliosis Spinal Twist Result

Short Leg

Long Leg

Injured Leg

Supporting Leg that does all the work

When you walk on one leg the foot must point outwards more to support all the weight. This makes the outside of the leg tighter which will pull the hips

24

backward and shift the pelvis to the injured leg side. This will affect the foundation of the spine and it will start to curve causing scoliosis. The spine will continue to curve all the way up the neck and cause cervical neck pain. So, if you have a chronic neck pain on the right side of the neck then you are not flexing your left toe (which would be the short leg). When one leg is shorter than the other it best just to concentrate on this shorter leg. Step Point 4 is best used to lengthen a short leg. This requires hitting the big toe and lengthening your leg behind you. If you work on these issues without flexing the toe, your symptoms of low back pain, hip pain and scoliosis will continually need to be treated.

If your injury has never been massaged you may find that the area may still have some hardness around it, and this is scar tissue. Massage techniques such as cross fiber friction, which is rubbing the opposite length of the muscle fibers, will help break up scar tissue bringing in circulation and cellular regeneration.

Fan Belt of Cause and Effect

When our foot transitions from Step Points 1-2 to Step Points 3-4, we are pushing on the outside of the foot transitioning to the inside foot. The fan belt analogy is showing that if one side is being tightened the other side is being pulled. Usually the side that is being pulled is where the pain is. Any appendage has a set of muscles that pull the appendage one way and then another set of muscles pull the appendage the opposite direction.

If we are walking on the outside of your feet only then you are tightening your IT Band (outside leg muscles) and straining/pulling your inside leg muscles. If you are standing on the back of your heels then you are straining the front of your legs. Both scenarios will lead to tight hips and symptoms like sciatica and low back pain occur.

To bring the fan belt of balance back inline one must flex the strained muscles. So, if you are used to walking on the outside of feet then you really need to focus on flexing your inside leg muscles when your leg is behind you.

The Fan Belt of Cause & Effect

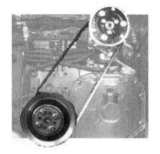

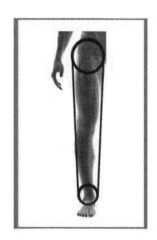

Cause		Effect
No Pain		Pain
Too Tight		Stretched
Knots		Strain
Greedy		Poor
Winning		Losing
Poor Technique		Shin Splints
Too Strong		Too Weak

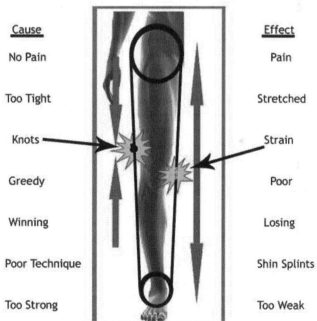

Toes pointed in & toes pointed out - Postural Affect

For a moment, try standing with your toes pointed outward. You may notice that you begin to fall backwards. To keep from falling backwards one must slightly curve their spine and head forward to counter the balance. People who walk or stand with their toes pointed outward will often report neck and mid-back pain due to stress on their spine.

If one followed Part 2 and kept their toes pointed forward, this posture would be prevented. When the toes are pointed forward for the whole leg stride, this will tilt the chest back and your skull will go backwards and firmly rest on top of your cervical spine.

When you walk on the outside of your feet it is very easy to combine Step Point 3 & 4 together at the same time. Take special notice to separate these Step Points and feel the inside of your thigh burn...then it is working.

Posture of people who walk with their toes pointed inward

When people walk with their toes pointed inward, they will start to fall forward. The front of their hips, thighs, and front of the calves will be tight from this incorrect walking technique. Since they are continually falling forward they may over arch their back which will tilt their hips forward causing low and mid back pain. Some Runners may fall into this category as the Running Technique is closely related to causing the same symptoms.

Walking with your toes pointed inwards may lead to ains on the inside of the legs or front of the hips.

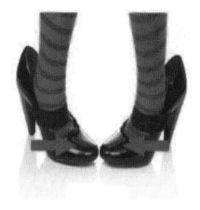
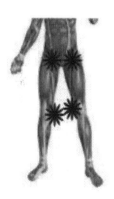

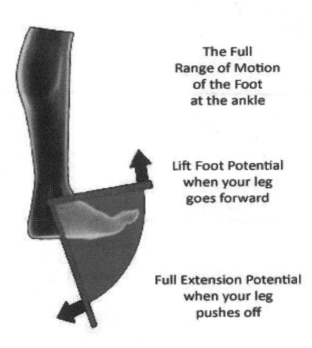

**The Full
Range of Motion
of the Foot
at the ankle**

**Lift Foot Potential
when your leg
goes forward**

**Full Extension Potential
when your leg
pushes off**

To help balance this posture one must focus more on the heel. Like in Part 1, lifting the foot more and make sure you really hit the heel and let your leg swing farther forward. It is also possible that Step Point 3 will be skipped as well. Make sure to hit all 4 Step Points separately and evenly.

Tip: Often inward toe walkers are stressed out and in a rush. I encourage these folks to slow down and take the time for themselves and get a massage.

Chapter 8

The Core

Engaging your Internal Muscles improves Posture

I have found that yoga instructors are very adamant about engaging your core. The core is your lower abdomen and hips. There is a lot of action that takes place here and being strong in your core is very important. In most yoga poses being strong in your cores helps with being able to hold some of the poses. The core helps you twist, stand up, and lift your legs. And of course, it is crucial to engage your core while walking.

Most yoga instructors will want you to engage your core while doing certain poses like chair and warrior pose. But the next step is focusing on your core with your inner legs at the same time. When walking, this action of engaging your core happens when your legs are apart like taking a walking stride or when doing the yoga warrior pose.

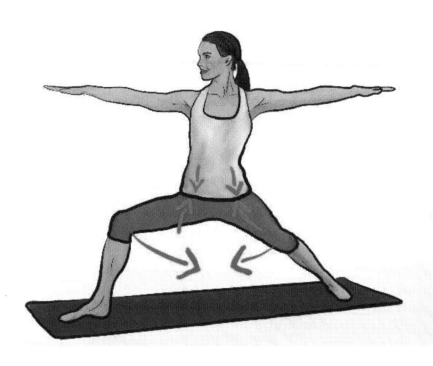

Warrior Pose

Most of the time bad posture starts with our bodies getting tired and we slump down into ourselves and slouch. Sometimes while driving in the morning I move my rearview mirror up and then by the evening I must move it down because I have shrunk throughout the day.

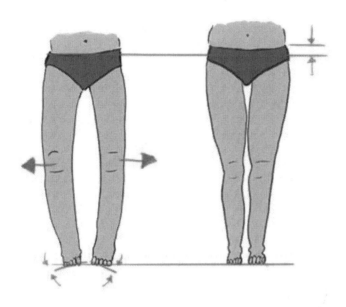

By engaging your core, you are helping to strengthen the inner muscle groups that hold you upright. I have noticed that there is a space between your hips and lower abdomen. I have noticed that my torso will slump into my hips. This in turn will bow my hip sockets out and my legs turn out and then I am walking on the outer edges of my feet. If I am strong in my core while engaging my inner legs, my torso lifts up and my feet become flat to the ground. I also notice my ankles have less pressure on them and if feels like I just lost 20 lbs. When we are off balance and have bad posture, our ankles and feet must make up for the imbalance. So, when you improve your posture, you will feel less pressure on your feet and ankles. Those that have ankle pain will want to pay special attention to this detail as it is likely your bad posture is creating your pain.

When we are in a bad posture and not engaging our core and not standing on our bones the muscles must make up the difference. Muscles do not like doing the job of bones. If the muscles do the skeletal work due to bad posture, they become very hard. I call this "bone tight" because your muscles become so tight they feel as hard as a bone.

Accessing your core does take some practice. It is a difficult concept to get at first. In yoga class, I heard the instructor talk about the core for years and for the longest time had no idea what they were talking about.

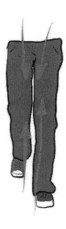

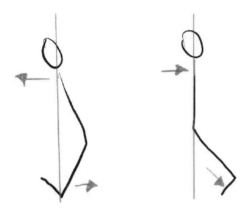

When you are about to access Step Point 3 (when stepping from Step Point 2 to 3), this is the point at which to engage the core of your inner hips and abdomen. When your leg is moving behind you, that is when you are flexing your inner leg and your core at the same time. Utilizing this technique will help push your shoulders and your head back into right alignment, which will give you a stronger upright posture.

Chapter 9:

Mental Manifesting

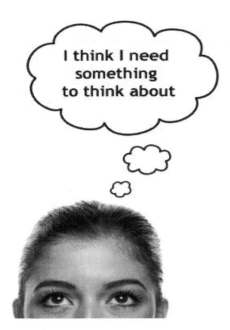

I think I need something to think about

As a Medical Intuitive, I have learned that the source of pain and disease starts in your mental interpretation of the world. The body's health is the direct result and reflection of your Mind's health. When the mind decides to create something, there is a specific process that happens from the initial identification of a problem all the way to a physical manifestation that remedies the situation. The same thing can be said about the technique of throwing a ball. If there is a problem with the throwing action somewhere, in the mind will be the same problem. A walking stride can exhibit the same pattern as the mind process. If one has a hiccup in the mind, the body will copy and express the same hiccup. So, pain and circumstance can reflect the same pattern you may be skipping in your mental manifestations.

In Part 3, I go over the 4 Stepping Points of the physical body. Really, I should start with the Mental Aspects of walking before the Physical aspects of walking. However, not a lot of people are ready to hear about the concept that they may be causing their own health demise. Also, if you want to put your health back on your terms, you are going to have to do your own research. I recommend getting multiple opinions for practitioners from different modalities. With the myriad of opinions, I read between the lines and choose what I am going to do. People would rather blame others and genetics for their health problems. I can confidently tell you from my experience it does hurt at first, but if you can accept this concept, that you create your health, then you will see so many life improvements occur. When you take responsibility for your own health, your life will go from boring and hopeless to purposeful and joyful. Putting all your faith in others exposes you to be a victim of your own ignorance.

By being able to observe how my body works, I have also been able to observe how my mind works and I have come up with these 4 Mental Step Points that correspond to the 4 Physical Step Points.

The 4 Mental Step Points:

1. Clear intention of dreams and desires.
2. Commit to Action.
3. Following Through.
4. Accepting the Outcome.

Steps 1 & 2 both work with developing a clear plan and then deciding to fulfill it, as it relates to current wants and needs. Steps 3-4 work with the "doing" of said intention and being responsible to see the plan and accepting the good with the bad. Once this action is complete, reflection upon the outcome will determine what needs to be done for next time.

Both techniques of the spiritual mind connecting with the body are crucial factors that must be looked at. Using one or the other is not enough. The sum will be added up in our overall physical and spiritual health. Every issue can be resolved if we focus on the physical symptoms and the mental issues. If the mind is the source of the pain, just taking care of the body may delay resolutions and the issue will come up again later.

Ideally, it is best to work with a variety of practitioners who work in different areas. A spiritual advisor or counselor is best for Spiritual and Mental guidance and on the physical level, herbs and manual therapies area also helpful. When you witness how each practitioner solves your issues then you can see the bigger part of the equation. If you only work with one practitioner or modality, then you may only see a small part of the big picture which may not make any sense.

In Part 2: Toes Forward - 80% of the People walk with their toes outward and then there is the 20% of people walk with their toes inward.

The Mental Aspect of the 80% outward toe walkers.

I have noticed a pattern within each group in their Mental Step Points. When you walk with your toes outward you will roll Step Points 3 & 4 together at the same time. Specifically, Step Point 4 is being skipped. This point must do with "Accepting the Outcome". When you have your toes pointed outward this means you really don't want to "get there". Sometimes when we find out we have been doing something wrong we go into denial and don't want to hear that we have been sabotaging a piece of ourselves for most of our life. It takes a lot of courage to be able to hear constructive criticism without becoming upset and taking it personally. What we should really be putting into our intention is, "I want to be the best at what I do, so I will listen to all possible aspects that I may be doing wrong." When you can listen to a coach or counselor giving you advice to improve your performance this will only enhance the outcome. The same goes with running a business, completing a project, or listening to your partner. By being open to hear guidance from others and hear the painful advice from your body, this will be the beginning of putting you on track for optimal health on your terms. Understanding how things truly work and then implementing them is the grand key to achieving enlightenment, soul purpose and pure bliss.

The Mental Aspect of the 20% inward toe walkers.

The other 20% that walk with their toes pointed inwards are skipping Step Points 1 & 2. They are running on their toes and not hitting the heel. These people are usually in a big rush and are always falling forward. Because they have not clearly stated their goals on what they specifically want, they have the feeling of always being behind. When you don't state your goals then you do a lot of extra running around hoping you run into them. They are also in such a rush and they will always overlook the opportunity because it has not manifested yet. One must be patient and allow your intention to manifest. It is a lot like throwing a ball; these people will throw the ball of intention and then expend all their energy to run to where the ball is landing. Then they get hit in the back of the head and they think that next time they just need to run faster. In fact, all they need to do is trust that they are playing catch with the universe and are supposed to throw the ball and let the universe throwback something better in return.

Inward toe walkers need to let that heel dig into the ground and SLOW DOWN. Be patient with where you are at because chasing your tail ends up in the same place that you started. Watch and you will see that by slowing down you will get more things done and will waste way less time and resources.

So instead of slamming the door on the unwanted house guest called pain, invite it in as a secret counsel for the next steps you need to take. Empowering ourselves and being responsible for our own lives brings clarity and purpose to living. We are shown everyday hints on how to lead our lives and pain is one those gifts. Embrace the messenger, and walk in peace.

Chapter 10:

The Bad & Ideal Shoes

Bad Shoes

As previously stated in Part 5, it is best to be able to feel the ground and fully flex your feet. In the waitress world, there is a popular shoe that most wear that is like a clog. The sole is very hard and the foot cannot flex into the ground. Many waitresses and servers have low back, hip, or leg issue. When waitresses change their shoes to a more flexible shoe, their issues cease within a week. Binding your feet or wearing too cushy of a sole does not help foot health either. Flexing and actively stretching your feet is best for circulation and structure strengthening.

Ideal Shoes

I like to wear Skechers, which are in my opinion, a sporty good-looking shoe. The sole is very thin and I can really feel the ground. Another Shoe company with a thin sole is Vibram, I like to call their shoes "Monkey Feet", and they look like gloves for your feet. This is the best shoe scenario because one will ultimately feel every piece of the ground and your feet will become very strong. However, one must start out slow because walking correctly at first is very hard. Pace yourself and work the Walking Series slowly.

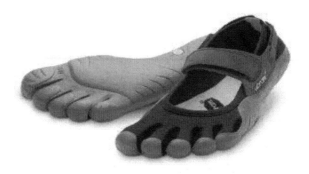

When I was in my teens, I was a competitive swimmer. After that I moved onto sports like running and softball. I developed very bad shin splints which is the direct result of walking on the outside of your feet. It took me two years to be able to walk correctly around Green Lake in Seattle which is about 3 miles long. I slowly built up to being able to walk that far. Breaking the bad habit of walking is mentally tough as well physically challenging.

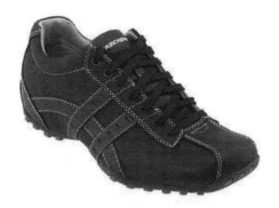

New Shoes

If you are going to start walking correctly you are going to
have to get some new shoes. Attempting to walk correctly
with your old shoes that are worn out is very difficult. As the
shoes wear out naturally the wear will continually get worse
and your walking technique also gets slowly worse. If you
walk on the outside of your feet, the heel and outside edge
becomes more and more worn and attempting to hit the
inside foot becomes harder to do. It feels like you have a
large bump in your shoe which make walking correctly
harder to maintain.

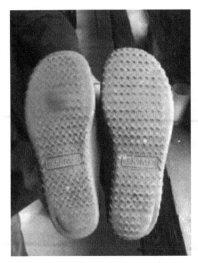 I have been able to observe my shoes lasting much longer now because I work my feet evenly on both sides. So not only will walking correctly help your leg joint health but will also help you from buying more shoes.

Tip: Walking barefoot over rocks is a fantastic way to massage and strengthen your feet.

Note the worn tread from leaning to the right side while walking. Also see the bottom outside heels are worn from pointing the toes outward.

Chapter 11:

Solutions & Exercises for Superior Walking Health

Walking Meditation

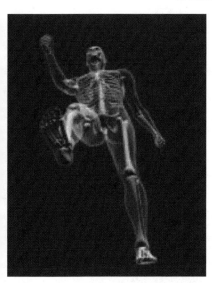

For all those over-thinkers who can't get out of their head, thinking about your feet is a great mediation exercise. When one thinks about how their feet touch the ground, it helps you forget about repetitive or useless thoughts. It's like you are sucking all the excess thoughts out of your head and using it as glue to connect with the Earth. If you really think about it, with all that thinking do you really get more done? Taking a break and feeling your body touch the earth, will help your conscious rest and your subconscious will come up with better ideas. Plus, when you take time to rest your body, the mind has a better house to settle in.

Massage Therapy

Massage is great for loosening very tight walking muscles. When you have been walking for decades incorrectly it is difficult to just go cold turkey and suddenly start successfully walking the correct way. Improper technique has become a habit and breaking habits takes some time to undo. After decades of walking incorrectly, overstretched muscles can be very difficult to engage. Overstretched muscles will usually be the muscles that are causing the pain. Flexing these muscles will keep them from becoming more stretched and once flexed they will stretch the over used tight muscles which exhibit no pain. "Typical toe outward" people will have tight outside legs and over stretched inside legs.

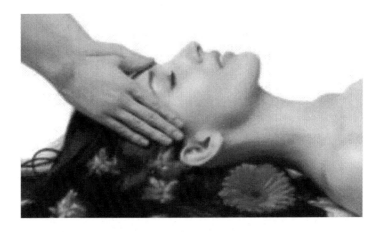

Massage can help get you started walking correctly because massage techniques such as cross fiber friction can help break up scar tissue in the muscles. Once these tight muscles can relax a bit it will be easier to flex and strengthen the overstretched muscles. "Knots" and "ropey" muscles are overstretched muscles. They have become this way because when a muscle is overstretched it must protect itself by hardening itself. The overstretched muscles are the ones that exude the pain because the tendon is about to be ripped from the bone. Tight muscles are the real cause which usually exudes no pain because they are stealing the space from the overstretched muscles. It is like a tug a war in your body. The best way to resolve the battle is to balance the scale. Flex overstretched muscles and stretch the tight ones. You can rub overstretched muscles all day and it will have very little lasting effect. By stretching and lengthening the tight muscle that gives off no pain, you will have more beneficial relief to the overstretched muscle.

Yoga: Chair Pose

There are not too many exercise for the inside legs besides walking but there is one that will let you know about your inside legs. The Chair Pose!

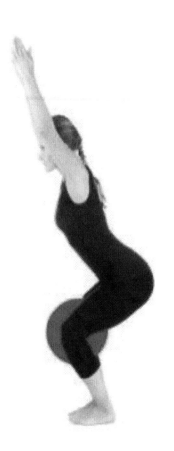

To really access the inside leg muscles, it is important to have a firm object in between your knees or thighs like a soft soccer ball, Yamana ball, firm pillow, yoga block, or a bouncy red ball.

Put the firm object between your knees and squeeze them tighter and strike the Chair Pose. Feel the inside legs burn and push your inside feet downwards into the ground.

It is important to feel these muscles as this will add more awareness to your walking technique and you will know if you are walking correctly or not. Step Point 3 & 4 is all inside legs and is imperative to a correct walking posture.

Chapter 12

The StretchFlex Technique™

A Stretch a day keeps the Surgeon away

The StretchFlex Technique™ can be overlaid onto any stretch that you already know and it just requires one more step.

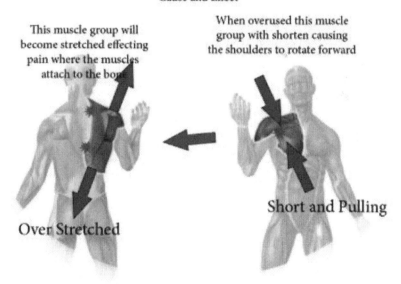

Opposing Muscle Groups
Cause and Effect

This muscle group will become stretched effecting pain where the muscles attach to the bone

When overused this muscle group with shorten causing the shoulders to rotate forward

Over Stretched

Short and Pulling

When you do a normal stretch notice where the pain is. The pain is the tight muscle being stretched. While you are at the end of the stretch, focus on precisely where the pain is located and then begin to flex that muscle in the opposite direction. Note: One always needs resistance to flex the muscle into something like an elastic band, door frame, bench, or friend holding your arm or leg. Flexing into the air sort-of works but it is best to flex into an item. It is an easy technique to do...to the observer it may look like you are just doing the traditional stretch. If you can do multiple slight little flexes and stretches you will notice significant improvements and have greater range of motion and less pain with any appendage.

Opposing Muscle Groups
Sharing the same appendage

This Muscle Group
Brings the Arm Backwards

This Muscle Group
Brings the Arm Forward

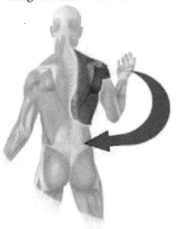
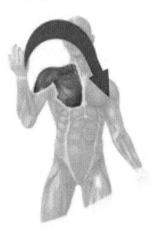

If you are doing the traditional hamstring stretch where you straighten your leg over bench...stretch the back of your hamstring and then keep your leg straight and flex the painful muscle downward into the bench. The same technique can be applied when stretching the Pectoral Chest muscle. Against a door frame, stretch your arm backwards and when you feel that is as far as you can stretch then flex the muscle forward focusing on flexing the painful chest muscle.

If your neck is overstretched, and most peoples are, while lying on a bed tuck your chin and flex your head backwards into the bed. This will shorten and strengthen the back of your neck muscles which will help one have fewer headaches.

The StretchFlex Technique™ will greatly improve your range of motion and you will have less pain doing it which will likely lead you to doing more stretches.

It is important to flex and stretch every appendage in both directions. Pain is usually from an over stretched muscle. However just focusing on over stretched muscles is only half the problem. By working both sides of the motion you will increase the integrity of that joint. This is often what Carpal Tunnel, Computer mouse arm, Headaches, and Arthritis is all about...the joint is being pulled too often in one direction and pain is the indicator that the appendage needs to be balanced.

In regard to How to Walk Correctly, the whole walking stride is the only time we are stretching and flexing. In Step Point 1 when you lift your foot before your heel hits the ground you are flexing the front of your shin (Tibialis Anterior Muscle), after Step Point 4 you are pushing off your toe and flexing your calf muscle. This action can be the StretchFlex Technique™. Also in the Step Point 1 you are opening your arch and between Step Point 2 and 3 you are then flexing your arch. When you are using Step Point 1 and 2 you are flexing your outside leg muscles and when you are using Step Point 3 and 4 you are using your inside leg muscles.

So, in a single stride you are using the StretchFlex Technique™ 3 times. Any lack of flexing in any of these areas will create all of the previous ailments that this book is about. Exercising the full range of motion in any appendage will help prevent and maintain all your joints.

Sometimes muscles can be so tight that they are not stretchable. A massage 2-4 times a month will help loosen that muscle and then the StretchFlex Technique™ will be easier to do.

Using the StretchFlex Technique™ may prevent Arthritis and any other potential injuries which will hopefully keep you off the operating table.

The StretchFlex Technique™ only requires about 2-5 minutes a day. After about 1-2 weeks you may notice some significant improvement. I think this technique is 10 times more effective than just stretching and is less painful.

By being aware of how to maintain your body and know when you are about to hurt yourself, which will lead to better health and overall greater spiritual awareness.

Pain is the body showing you how to heal yourself – Pain Awareness. Often stretching is associated with pain which is probably the reason why many don't do it. But if you flex the pain, you are putting awareness back into your body and awareness in and of itself reduces pain.

<u>Conclusion</u>

So, as you can see there is a lot going on in every step we take. Taking our time to pay attention to all the tiny aspects of our life can start to explain what is going on in life. Reflecting on how you live your life and slowing it down, we can then start to diagnose what we are doing right and wrong. I believe there are solutions everywhere and that most world, personal, and relationship problems can be solved. Typically, they are so simple that it is unfathomable. I hope this super detail focus of How to Walk Correctly will help you with your walk and perhaps see that if you slow the world down a little bit you can be responsible for yourself and empower your own healing.

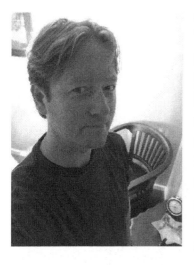

Jacob Caldwell is a Massage Therapist in Seattle. He is passionate about how to help people address the issues they have and will help those that want to heal themselves. In this complex world simplicity is being lost. Jacob has found most of the solutions in the world are quite easy. He is on a mission to help assist in making the world simple.

Walking Correctly can't be any easier, which is the hard part.

www.SeattleMassageBlogger.com

www.SeattleMasssage.co

www.EnergyHealingTherapy.net

Instagram "how2walkcorrectly"

Facebook Fanpage "Seattle Massage Therapy"

Other Books
Authored & Illustrated
by
Jacob Caldwell

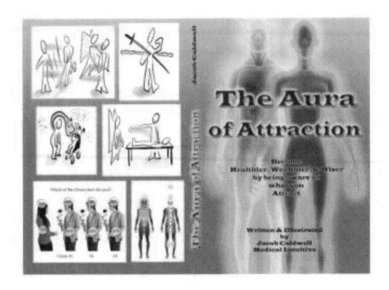

Take the Aura of Attraction Survey
to see what you Attract
Facebook Fanpage "The Aura of Attraction"

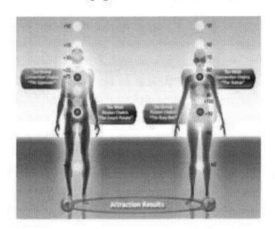

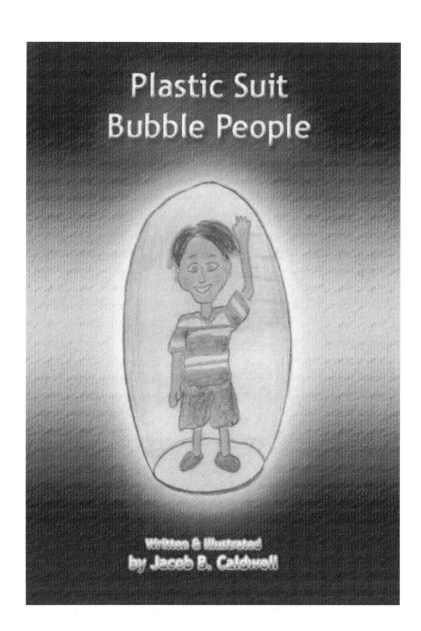

Book Description

This guide on How to Walk Correctly is for people who want to be responsible for their own healing. This step by step process of walking correctly will help you alleviate your own leg issues. This is one of the ways to never have to be in a wheel chair or the need to wear orthotics. Walking Correctly will help your overall posture and many of your leg, back, and neck chronic issues may be able to lessen or disappear.

Jacob Caldwell is a Massage Therapist in Seattle who will assist you in empowering you to heal yourself. He has over 15 years of experience in helping people see that you can alleviate your own symptoms by just Walking Correctly.

Continuing Education for Health Practitioners

Instructor: Jacob Caldwell, LMP

MA000016444

Steps2Light@yahoo.com

Seattle, WA 98199

"How to Walk Correctly" Book   **2 Hours of CEU**

CEU's are for reading this book.

Homework: Apply the lessons to yourself and then to your clients.

Make a copy for your CEU records or tear from the book. Keep a receipt for your records.

Student_____ MA_____ Date_____

Made in the USA
Columbia, SC
10 September 2023